GOD'S WAY OUT OF OLD AGE

Discover God's way of making you younger.

Note: All scripture are quoted from www.biblegateway.com

TABLE OF CONTENTS

INTRODUCTION
Old age sets in immediately when a person is born. As the days count, so the body gravitates towards getting old and starts to wear out. Someone has to fight to keep it younger long enough for it hosts the real you. We see our parents, aunts, uncles and grandparents having bodies that we don't admire but the reality hits us that even we are headed there. They are the image of where we

are headed only that they arrived early. Most people have a problem accepting this reality that their days on earth are reducing and their bodies are losing strength faster than they can track. The fear of old age,thoughts of death, rejection, inability to achieve dreams set in. The attitude changes from that of celebrating life to wishing for the young days. Time flies so fast that any birthday is just a reminder of how little time remaining on earth is getting. Emotions of jealousy sets in when someone sees young people. Moreso, when you see them wasting their time and any advice given they don't take. They see they are young and time is on their side but as for you their presence is a reminder of the good old days and how you wasted them just like they are doing. Now you have gained a little wisdom out of experience and though experience they say it's the best teacher, you wish you knew earlier how to number your days.

Psalms 90:9-12
For all our days have passed away in Your wrath;
We finish our years like a sigh.
The days of our lives are seventy years;
And if by reason of strength they are eighty years,
Yet their boast is only labour and sorrow;
For it is soon cut off, and we fly away.

Who knows the power of Your anger?
For as the fear of You, so is Your wrath.
So teach us to number our days,
That we may gain a heart of wisdom

The good news is that there is a way out of the fear of old age.
When all seems to be beyond our control, God is ever in control
and he has a way out of old age into long life and being younger.

1st corinthians 10:13
No temptation has overtaken you except such as is common to
man; but God is faithful, who will not allow you to be tempted
beyond what you are able, but with the temptation **will also make
the way of escape**, that you may be able to bear it.

However, the ways of God are opposite the ways of the world.
Therefore, his way to being young may not agree with your mind
but you walk with God by faith not by sight.

Romans 12:2
Do not conform to the pattern of this world, but be transformed by
the renewing of your mind. Then you will be able to test and
approve what God's will is—his good, pleasing and perfect will.

You agree with his word not what the world is saying. That's the only way to please him so that you receive the reward of being younger.

2nd corinthians 5:7
For we walk by faith, not by sight.

Hebrews 11:6
And without faith it is impossible to please God, because anyone who comes to him must believe that he exists and that he rewards those who earnestly seek him.

CHAPTER ONE: IN.THE BEGINNING
Everything starts from the beginning.

Genesis 1:1
In the beginning God created the heaven and the earth.

When God created the earth, there was no old age. He created Adam in his image and likeness and he is full of life.

Genesis 1:26-27

Then God said, "Let Us make man in Our image, according to Our
likeness; let them have dominion over the fish of the sea, over the
birds of the air, and over the cattle, over all the earth and over
every creeping thing that creeps on the earth." So God created
man in His own image; in the image of God He created him; male
and female He created them.

John 1:4
In Him was life, and the life was the light of men.

Adam was to eat from the tree of life. He was like God and eating
from the tree of life brought life to his body.

Genesis 2:8-9
The Lord God planted a garden eastward in Eden, and there He put
the man whom He had formed. And out of the ground the Lord
God made every tree grow that is pleasant to the sight and good for
food. ***The tree of life was also in the midst of the garden,*** and the
tree of the knowledge of good and evil.

Old age was never God's will but choices have consequences. God
didn't create a robot but a human being with free will. He advised

Adam not eat from the tree of good and evil for that would open a door to death.

Genesis 2:16-17
And the Lord God commanded the man, saying, "Of every tree of the garden you may freely eat; _**but of the tree of the knowledge of good and evil you shall not eat, for in the day that you eat of it you shall surely die."**_

God knew an angel had rebelled and thrown out of heaven and was out to destroy all that God had made. Satan was his name and that instruction was to protect Adam from getting the same thing the fallen angel got, death. God is life, when Satan chose to disconnect himself from him, he became the author of death.

Revelation 12:7-9
And war broke out in heaven: Michael and his angels fought with the dragon; and the dragon and his angels fought, but they did not prevail, nor was a place found for them in heaven any longer. **So the great dragon was cast out, that serpent of old, called the Devil and Satan, who deceives the whole world; he was cast to the earth, and his angels were cast out with him.**

The option presented before Adam was either to feed from the tree of life and receive more life from God or feed from the tree of good and evil and receive death from satan. The love of God for Adam wanted him to choose life but his love also grants freedom to choose but the consequences are inevitable.

Deuteronomy 30:19
I call heaven and earth as witnesses today against you, that **I have set before you life and death**, blessing and cursing; **therefore choose life, that both you and your descendants may live.**

When Satan proposed the idea of eating from the tree of good and evil, Adam believed it. Satan did not show them the consequences of eating from the tree of good and evil, he lied to them that there were benefits that God didn't tell them of.

John 8:44
You belong to your father, the devil, and you want to carry out your father's desires. He was a murderer from the beginning, not holding to the truth, for there is no truth in him. When he lies, he speaks his native language, for he is a liar and the father of lies.

He chose to disobey God and ate from the tree that brought death and old age was part of the package. Even if it was God's desire that Adam should eat from the tree of life, Adam by his own free will, chose to eat from the tree of good and evil and he inherited all Satan had.

Genesis 3: 1-7

Now the serpent was more cunning than any beast of the field which the Lord God had made. And he said to the woman, "Has God indeed said, 'You shall not eat of every tree of the garden'?" And the woman said to the serpent, "We may eat the fruit of the trees of the garden; but of the fruit of the tree which is in the midst of the garden, God has said, 'You shall not eat it, nor shall you touch it, lest you die.' "

Then the serpent said to the woman, "You will not surely die. For God knows that in the day you eat of it your eyes will be opened, and you will be like God, knowing good and evil."

So when the woman saw that the tree was good for food, that it was pleasant to the eyes, and a tree desirable to make one wise, she took off its fruit and ate. **She also gave to her husband with her, and he ate. Then the eyes of both of them were opened, and they knew that they were naked;** and they sewed fig leaves together and made themselves coverings.

This is why it's important to trust the Love of God that when he says keep off from something, he is a loving father and knows why he said that. Trust in a relationship with God is important. You trust who you love. Be established in God's love that you will trust every command he gives. If Adam had known the love of God, he would have trusted his command and would not have bought into the lies of satan.

Jude 1:21
keep yourselves in the love of God.

Ephesians 3:17-19
that Christ may dwell in your hearts through faith; **that you, _being rooted and grounded in love_, may be able to comprehend with all the saints what is the width and length and depth and height, to know the love of Christ which passes knowledge; that you may be filled with all the fullness of God.**

Eve on the other side represents believers who are ignorant. There are so many things that God had said and done that she didn't know and there are things God had not said that she added. Ignorance is another ground Satan takes advantage of among the children of God.

Hosea 4:6
my people are destroyed from lack of knowledge.

Therefore, seek to know the word of God and his love so that you will stand against all that Satan throws at you.

2nd corinthians 2:11
Lest Satan should get an advantage of us: for we are not ignorant of his devices.

1st john 2:15-17
Do not love the world or the things in the world. If anyone loves the world, the love of the Father is not in him. For all that is in the world—the lust of the flesh, the lust of the eyes, and the pride of life—is not of the Father but is of the world. And the world is passing away, and the lust of it; but he who does the will of God abides forever.

From that time, all men from Adam started becoming old and finally when their bodies were worn out completely, their spirits left.

Romans 5:12
Therefore, just as through one man sin entered the world, and death through sin, and thus **death spread to all men,** because all sinned.

God is a spirit and he breathed himself into Adam. Spirits live forever like God lives forever. The body just hosts the spirits but when time comes to leave the body, the spirits are hosted forever either in heaven or hell. The choice to follow God or Satan is still open today. Adam chose satan and opened the door for death to set in that affected all human beings. That was how old age stepped in the world and its effect is being seen until today.

Romans 5:14
Nevertheless death reigned from Adam to Moses, even over those who had not sinned according to the likeness of the transgression of Adam, who is a type of Him who was to come.

CHAPTER TWO: THE NEW BEGINNING

God is love and he had a plan of introducing the tree of life back to humanity. He did that by sending his only begotten son, Jesus. He came as the life of God.

John 3:16

For God so loved the world that He gave His only begotten Son, that whoever believes in Him should not perish but have _everlasting life._

Jesus chose to obey God and went to the cross where he took the curse of old age on his body and when he rose from the dead, he became the tree of life for those who chose him.

John 15:1

I am the true vine, and My Father is the vinedresser.

Adam fell by eating, Jesus introduced a new way of eating. Jesus said he was the tree of life and his body and blood were the new diet to being younger.

John 6:50-51

This is the bread which comes down from heaven, ***that one may eat of it and not die.*** **I am the living bread which came down from heaven. If anyone eats of this bread, he will live forever;** and the bread that I shall give is My flesh, which I shall give for the life of the world."

Adams eating from the tree of good and evil brought in death, but eating from the body of Jesus who is the tree of life brings in life and being young is part of that package.

John 6:53-57

Then Jesus said to them, "Most assuredly, I say to you, unless you eat the flesh of the Son of Man and drink His blood, you have no life in you. Whoever eats My flesh and drinks My blood has eternal life, and I will raise him up at the last day. For My flesh is food indeed, and My blood is drink indeed. He who eats My flesh and drinks My blood abides in Me, and I in him. As the living Father sent Me, and I live because of the Father, so he who feeds on Me will live because of Me.

The ways of God are so simple it takes people to complicate them.
Also, the ways of God are so foolish that if you don't choose them
from your spirit, your fallen mind will reject them.
The choice is still presented before you which tree you will feed
from. Will you feed from the tree of life who is Christ or will you
feed from the tree of good and evil which is the world.

1st corinthians 27-29
But God has chosen the foolish things of the world to put to shame
the wise, and God has chosen the weak things of the world to put
to shame the things which are mighty; and the base things of the
world and the things which are despised God has chosen, and the
things which are not, to bring to nothing the things that are, that no
flesh should glory in His presence.

It was Jesus who introduced the holy communion. He taught us
how to take the Lord's body and blood and that opened a door for
us to life.

Mathew 26:26-28
And as they were eating, Jesus took bread, blessed and broke it,
and gave it to the disciples and said, ***"Take, eat; this is My body."***

Then He took the cup, and gave thanks, and gave it to them,
saying, "Drink from it, all of you. For this is My blood of the new
covenant, which is shed for many for the remission of sins.

Today, Jesus is our second Adam. As he is young in heaven, so
will we be down here on earth when we eat his body and blood.
When we believe in Jesus, we have a new beginning.

2nd corinthians 5:17
Therefore, if anyone is in Christ, he is a new creation; the old has
passed away, and see, the new has come!

The Lord Jesus himself took the body and blood and gave it to his
disciples who had not recognized him while he walked physically
with them. After they ate, he vanished from their site. That's how
he wants you to know his ways, through the word and through
seeing his body on the cross hanged there for you to have access to
life, health, joy, peace etc.

Luke 24:13-35
ke 24:13-35

Now that same day two of them were going to a village called
Emmaus, about seven miles from Jerusalem. They were talking
with each other about everything that had happened. As they talked
and discussed these things with each other, Jesus himself came up
and walked along with them; but they were kept from recognizing
him.
He asked them, "What are you discussing together as you walk
along?"

They stood still, their faces downcast. One of them, named
Cleopas, asked him, "Are you the only one visiting Jerusalem who
does not know the things that have happened there in these days?"
 "What things?" he asked.

"About Jesus of Nazareth," they replied. "He was a prophet,
powerful in word and deed before God and all the people. The
chief priests and our rulers handed him over to be sentenced to
death, and they crucified him; but we had hoped that he was the
one who was going to redeem Israel. And what is more, it is the
third day since all this took place. In addition, some of our women
amazed us. They went to the tomb early this morning but didn't
find his body. They came and told us that they had seen a vision of
angels, who said he was alive. Then some of our companions went

to the tomb and found it just as the women had said, but they did not see Jesus.”

He said to them, “How foolish you are, and how slow to believe all that the prophets have spoken! Did not the Messiah have to suffer these things and then enter his glory?” And beginning with Moses and all the Prophets, he explained to them what was said in all the Scriptures concerning himself.

As they approached the village to which they were going, Jesus continued on as if he were going farther. But they urged him strongly, “Stay with us, for it is nearly evening; the day is almost over.” So he went in to stay with them.

When he was at the table with them, he took bread, gave thanks, broke it and began to give it to them. Then their eyes were opened and they recognized him, and he disappeared from their sight. They asked each other, “Were not our hearts burning within us while he talked with us on the road and opened the Scriptures to us?”

They got up and returned at once to Jerusalem. There they found the Eleven and those with them, assembled together and saying, “It is true! The Lord has risen and has appeared to Simon.” Then the two told what had happened on the way, and how Jesus was recognized by them when he broke the bread.

Choose to believe that as you eat the body and drink the blood of Jesus that paid for the long life, health and young age you desire, your body will be like the body of Jesus. There is no old age in Jesus and so old age will not be found in you. Many believers are experiencing the effects of the curse of old age for they are not taking the body of Jesus and those who do, take it religiously without revelation.

1st Corinthians 11:17-34
 Now in giving these instructions I do not praise you, since you come together not for the better but for the worse. For first of all, when you come together as a church, I hear that there are divisions among you, and in part I believe it. For there must also be factions among you, that those who are approved may be recognized among you. Therefore when you come together in one place, it is not to eat the Lord's Supper. For in eating, each one takes his own supper ahead of others; and one is hungry and another is drunk. What! Do you not have houses to eat and drink in? Or do you despise the church of God and shame those who have nothing? What shall I say to you? Shall I praise you in this? I do not praise you.

For I received from the Lord that which I also delivered to you: **that the Lord Jesus on the same night in which He was betrayed took bread; and when He had given thanks, He broke it and said, "Take, eat; this is My body which is broken for you; do this in remembrance of Me."** In the same manner He also took the cup after supper, saying, "This cup is the new covenant in My blood. This do, as often as you drink it, in remembrance of Me."
For as often as you eat this bread and drink this cup, you proclaim the Lord's death till He comes.
 Therefore whoever eats this bread or drinks this cup of the Lord in an unworthy manner will be guilty of the body and blood of the Lord. But let a man examine himself, and so let him eat of the bread and drink of the cup. **For he who eats and drinks in an unworthy manner eats and drinks judgement to himself, not discerning the Lord's body. For this reason many are weak and sick among you, and many sleep.** For if we would judge ourselves, we would not be judged. But when we are judged, we are chastened by the Lord, *that we may not be condemned with the world.*
Therefore, my brethren, when you come together to eat, wait for one another. But if anyone is hungry, let him eat at home, lest you

come together for judgement. And the rest I will set in order when
I come.

CHAPTER THREE: EAT YOUR WAY TO BEING YOUNGER
The children of Israel are a shadow of the church. We who are in
Christ have the real thing. We can learn from the children of Isreal
who were in the old covenant and experienced access to being
young. We are in a better covenant therefore our lives should be
better.

Colosians 2:16-17
So let no one judge you in food or in drink, or regarding a festival
or a new moon or sabbaths, which are a shadow of things to come,
but the substance is of Christ.

Hebrews 8:6
But now He has obtained a more excellent ministry, inasmuch as
He is also Mediator of a better covenant, which was established on
better promises.

Romans 15:4

For whatever things were written before were written for our learning, that we through the patience and comfort of the Scriptures might have hope.

The children of Israel were slaves for 430 years. A slave doesn't eat well, they were subjected to hard labour, they didn't have the privileges of taking care of their bodies.

Exodus 5:10-19

Then the [Egyptian] taskmasters [in charge] of the people and their [Hebrew] foremen went out and said to the people, "Thus says Pharaoh, 'I will not give you any straw. Go, get straw for yourselves wherever you can find it, but your work [quota] will not be reduced in the least.'" So the people were scattered throughout the land of Egypt to gather stubble to use for straw. And the taskmasters pressured them, saying, "Finish your work, [fulfil] your daily quotas, just as when there was straw [given to you]." **And the Hebrew foremen, whom Pharaoh's taskmasters had set over them, were beaten and were asked, "Why have you not fulfilled your required quota of making bricks yesterday and today, as before?"** Then the Hebrew foremen came to Pharaoh and cried, "Why do you deal like this with your servants? No straw is given to your

servants, yet they say to us, 'Make bricks!' And look, your
servants are being beaten, but it is the fault of your own people."
But Pharaoh said, "You are lazy, very lazy and idle! That is why
you say, 'Let us go and sacrifice to the Lord.' Get out now and get
to work; for no straw will be given to you, yet you are to deliver
the same quota of bricks." The Hebrew foremen saw that they
were in a bad situation because they were told, "You must not
reduce [in the least] your daily quota of bricks."

However, the night they ate the lamb as God instructed, they came
out of Egypt so strong and none was feeble among them. That's the
power of eating the body of Christ.

Exodus 12:3-11
Speak to all the congregation of Israel, saying: 'On the tenth of this
month every man shall take for himself a lamb, according to the
house of his father, a lamb for a household. And if the household is
too small for the lamb, let him and his neighbour next to his house
take it according to the number of the persons; according to each
man's need you shall make your count for the lamb. Your lamb
shall be without blemish, a male of the first year. You may take it
from the sheep or from the goats. Now you shall keep it until the
fourteenth day of the same month. Then the whole assembly of the

congregation of Israel shall kill it at twilight. And they shall take some of the blood and put it on the two doorposts and on the lintel of the houses where they eat it. **Then they shall eat the flesh on that night; roasted in fire, with unleavened bread and with bitter herbs they shall eat it. Do not eat it raw, nor boiled at all with water, but roasted in fire—its head with its legs and its entrails.** You shall let none of it remain until morning, and what remains of it until morning you shall burn with fire. And **thus you shall eat it:** with a belt on your waist, your sandals on your feet, and your staff in your hand. So you shall eat it in haste. **It is the Lord's Passover.**

In the wilderness, no hotels neither houses to live in but only tents and Manna. They ate manna, the food of angels and their bodies never grew old.
There were those who despised the manna that God gave them and they died in the wilderness.

Psalms 78: 25-33
Man did eat angels' food (manna): he sent them meat to the full.

He caused an east wind to blow in the heaven: and by his power
he brought in the south wind.
He rained flesh also upon them as dust, and feathered fowls like as
the sand of the sea:
And he let it fall in the midst of their camp, round about their
habitations.
So they did eat, and were well filled: for he gave them their own
desire;
They were not estranged from their lust. But while their meat was
yet in their mouths,
The wrath of God came upon them, and slew the fattest of them,
and smote down the chosen men of Israel.
For all this they sinned still, and believed not for his wondrous
works.
Therefore their days did he consume in vanity, and their years in
trouble.

John 6:58
This is the bread which came down from heaven—not as your
fathers ate the manna, and are dead. He who eats this bread will
live forever."

Deuteronomy 8:3-4

So He humbled you, allowed you to hunger, and **fed you with manna** which you did not know nor did your fathers know, that He might make you know that man shall not live by bread alone; but man lives by every word that proceeds from the mouth of the Lord. **Your garments did not wear out on you, nor did your foot swell these forty years.**

But there were those like Caleb who valued this heavenly food and had access to long life and being young. There was no difference to Caleb when he was forty years and when he was eighty five years. His body had just been kept the same way by the power of God.
While Moses was lamenting that eighty years was how far those who rebelled in the wilderness went, he himself died at 120 years with his eyes so strong.

Deuteronomy 34:7
Moses was a hundred and twenty years old when he died, yet his eyes were not weak nor his strength gone.

Caleb on the other side became stronger as his days went, he lived so long that the bible does not record his death.

Joshua 14:6-15

 Then the children of Judah came unto Joshua in Gilgal: and Caleb
the son of Jephunneh the Kenezite said unto him, Thou knowest
the thing that the Lord said unto Moses the man of God concerning
me and thee in Kadesh Barnea.

 **Forty years old was I when Moses the servant of the Lord sent
me from Kadeshbarnea to espy out the land; and I brought
him word again as it was in mine heart.**

 Nevertheless my brethren that went up with me made the heart of
the people melt: but I wholly followed the Lord my God.

 And Moses sware on that day, saying, Surely the land whereon thy
feet have trodden shall be thine inheritance, and thy children's for
ever, because thou hast wholly followed the Lord my God.

**And now, behold, the Lord hath kept me alive, as he said, these
forty and five years, even since the Lord spake this word unto
Moses, while the children of Israel wandered in the wilderness:
and now, lo, I am this day fourscore and five years old (85
years).**

 _**As yet I am as strong this day as I was in the day that Moses sent
me: as my strength was then, even so is my strength now, for
war, both to go out, and to come in.**_

Now therefore give me this mountain, whereof the Lord spake in that day; for thou hearest in that day how the Anakims were there, and that the cities were great and fenced: if so be the Lord will be with me, then I shall be able to drive them out, as the Lord said. And Joshua blessed him, and gave unto Caleb the son of Jephunneh Hebron for an inheritance.

Hebron therefore became the inheritance of Caleb the son of Jephunneh the Kenezite unto this day, because that he wholly followed the Lord God of Israel.

And the name of Hebron before was Kirjatharba; which Arba was a great man among the Anakims. And the land had rest from war.

As you eat from the tree of life, the choice of how long you want to live will be up to you for God's power will keep you as long as you desire afterall, there is no time limit with God.

Deuteronomy 33:25
as thy days, so shall thy strength be.

CONCLUSION

The difference is in believing. Those who choose to believe God's ways get God's results but those who choose to believe the world way get the world's results. The world's way is Satan's way. He works opposite of how God works.

Jeremiah 6:16
Thus saith the Lord: "Stand ye in the highways and see, and ask for the old paths, where is the good way; and walk therein, and ye shall find rest for your souls. But they said, 'We will not walk therein.'

There is a lot of advice the world will give you on how to stay younger, but you can choose God's simple way and live. The choice still stands, and it's up to you to decide which side you are on. God loves you and has made the provisions for young age available for you. The choice however is yours.

2nd corinthians 11:3
But I fear lest by any means, as the serpent beguiled Eve through his subtlety, **so your minds should be corrupted from the simplicity that is in Christ.**

There is nothing glamorous about eating the body and the blood of Jesus represented by a piece of bread, biscuit, cake and water or juice but the power of God rests there.

Romans 1:16
For I am not ashamed of the gospel, because it is the power of God that brings salvation to everyone who believes: first to the Jew, then to the Gentile.

Make a decision to partake of the Lord's body and blood either alone or with family, friends, church members etc and watch the power of God start working in your body, keeping you younger and younger.
As you partake of the body and blood, see that curse of old age placed by God on the body of Jesus and as you behold him, the power of the holy spirit in you will make the life of God work in you.

2nd corinthians 3:18
But we all, with uncovered face beholding as in a glass the glory of the Lord, are changed into the same image, from glory to glory, even as by the Spirit of the Lord.

Old age is part of the curse that fell on humanity when Adam fell and chose satan but being younger is part of the blessing that comes on you when you believe in Jesus who chose to obey God.

Romans 5:15
But the free gift is not like the offence. For if by the one man's offence many died, **much more the grace of God and the gift by the grace of the one Man, Jesus Christ, abounded to many.**

Your youth will be renewed like the eagle. The eagle when it's old goes into the mountain and plucks all it's feathers, nails and beak. It's a tough process but when it endures, new feathers, nails and beak come out and it has a brand new life ahead of it.

Psalms 103:1-5
 Bless the Lord, O my soul;
And all that is within me, bless His holy name!
Bless the Lord, O my soul,
And forget not all His benefits:
Who forgives all your iniquities,
Who heals all your diseases,

Who redeems your life from destruction,
Who crowns you with lovingkindness and tender mercies,
Who satisfies your mouth with good things(Lord's body),
So that your youth is renewed like the eagle's.

As you partake of the body, stay at it. Don't give up halfway because you don't see results. Be patient and disciplined and with time you will see the changes in your physical body. The results God gives are so real that even those on the outside will tell you something is different about your body. When that happens, remember to give God all the glory.

Hebrews 10:35-39
Cast not away therefore your confidence, which hath great recompense of reward.
For ye have need of patience, that, after ye have done the will of God, ye might receive the promise.
"For yet a little while, and He that shall come will come, and will not tarry.
Now the just shall live by faith; but if any man draw back, My soul shall have no pleasure in him."
But we are not of those who draw back unto perdition, but of those who believe, to the saving of the soul.

JOHN 13:17
NOW THAT YOU KNOW THESE THINGS, YOU WILL BE
BLESSED IF YOU DO THEM.

More Grace on you as you eat your way to being younger to the
glory of God.

If you need help to study the word of God, email me at
pstmaryjoy@gmail.com and I will guide you through.

To get my other books in amazon, click this link
https://www.amazon.com/author/marynyandia